Farès Azaiez

Sport and anticoagulants

Farès Azaiez

Sport and anticoagulants

Approaches, Risks and Recommendations

ScienciaScripts

This book is a translation from the original published under ISBN 978-620-6-72485-8.

Publisher:
Sciencia Scripts
is a trademark of
Dodo Books Indian Ocean Ltd. and OmniScriptum S.R.L publishing group

120 High Road, East Finchley, London, N2 9ED, United Kingdom
Str. Armeneasca 28/1, office 1, Chisinau MD-2012, Republic of Moldova, Europe
Printed at: see last page
ISBN: 978-620-8-18943-3

TABLE OF CONTENTS

INTRODUCTION

Regular physical activity is recommended because of its recognised benefits in terms of reducing overall cardiovascular risk and preventing the development of several chronic diseases (1,2). On the other hand, a sedentary lifestyle is one of the main cardiovascular risk factors (3). Furthermore, coronary patients benefit from the effects of physical activity, which is a relevant aspect of secondary prevention of ischaemic disease (4).

In fact, physical activity has begun to be seen as part of the optimal therapy for patients, which is why it is now prescribed as a "drug" (5).

As a result, the widespread practice of physical activity involves people of all ages, both as a leisure activity and as a competitive sport.

Although these subjects are generally healthier than their peers with sedentary lifestyles, they are also at risk of a number of diseases, some of which are age-related and some of which require anticoagulant treatment.

The ultimate aim of sports participation in athletes at risk of bleeding is therefore to ensure that the benefits outweigh the harms.

In the present study, a review of the literature was used to establish the definition of an athlete and sporting activities, the various pathologies requiring anticoagulant treatment in athletes, and ways of managing this treatment in this category of patients.

REVIEW OF LITERATURE

I.   DEFINITION OF AN ATHLETE

The European Society of Cardiology (ESC) defines an athlete as "a person of young or adult age, amateur or professional, who trains regularly and takes part in official sports competitions" (6,7).

Similarly, the American Heart Association (AHA) defines a competitive athlete as a person involved in regular (usually intense) training in organised individual or team sports, with an emphasis on competition and performance (8,9).

By way of distinction, a recreational athlete plays sports for pleasure and leisure, whereas a competitive athlete is highly skilled and places greater emphasis on performance and winning.

In a proposed classification of athletes based on minimum volume of exercise, "elite" athletes (national team, Olympic and professional athletes) generally exercise ≥ 10h / week; "competitive" athletes [i.e. high school, college and older club] exercise
≥ 6 h / week; and recreational athletes exercise ≥ 4 h / week (10).

This distinction is somewhat arbitrary since some recreational athletes, such as long-distance cyclists and runners, can exercise at higher volumes than some professional athletes participating in skill sports.

II.   DEFINITION OF PHYSICAL EXERCISE

Although exercise and physical activity are often used interchangeably, it is important to recognise that these terms differ.

Physical activity is defined as any bodily movement produced by skeletal muscle that results in energy expenditure.

Exercise or exercise training, by definition, is a structured, repetitive physical activity designed to improve or maintain one or more components of physical fitness (11).

II.1 Characteristics of physical exercise

The basic principles of exercise prescription have been described using the "FITT" concept (frequency, intensity, time, and type). The mode of exercise is also an important characteristic.

II.1.1 -Frequency

The frequency of physical exercise is generally expressed as the number of times an individual exercises per week.

II.1.2 -Intensity

Of all the basic elements of exercise prescription, exercise intensity is generally considered to be the most important for achieving aerobic capacity and to have the most favourable impact on risk factors (12,13).

Absolute intensity refers to the rate of energy expenditure during exercise and is generally expressed in kcal/min or metabolic equivalents (METs) (14,15).

Relative exercise intensity refers to a fraction of an individual's maximum power (load) that is maintained during exercise and is generally prescribed as a percentage of maximal aerobic capacity (VO2max) on the basis of a cardiopulmonary exercise test (15).

Training intensity can also be expressed as a percentage of the maximum heart rate (HRmax) recorded during an exercise test (16) or predicted on the basis of the equation [HRmax = 220 - age] (17).

Alternatively, exercise intensity can be expressed in terms of a percentage of a person's HR reserve, which takes a percentage of the difference between HRmax and resting HR and adds it to the resting HR (Karvonen formula) (18).

II.1.3 -Time

The frequency and duration of training sessions provide the total energy expenditure of a training programme.

Compliance with the minimum activity guidelines is equivalent to around 1000 kcal/week or around 10 METs/hour/week.

The volume of training should increase each week either by 2.5% in intensity, or by 2 minutes, although the rate of progression should be individualised according to the individual's biological adaptation (19).

II.1.4 -Type

Different types of exercise are possible: coordination and balance, endurance, strength or resistance training, speed, flexibility.

II.1.5 -Mode

. Depending on metabolic expenditure: aerobic or anaerobic training

. Depending on the type of muscle work: isometric or isotonic, dynamic or static, continuous or intermittent, number of muscle groups involved.

II.2 Classification of sports

With regard to the choice of the most suitable sport, the doctor can indicate the type of sport as illustrated in figure 1 (skill, power, mixed or endurance), with specification of the frequency, duration and intensity of muscular work to be maintained preferentially during the exercise programme.

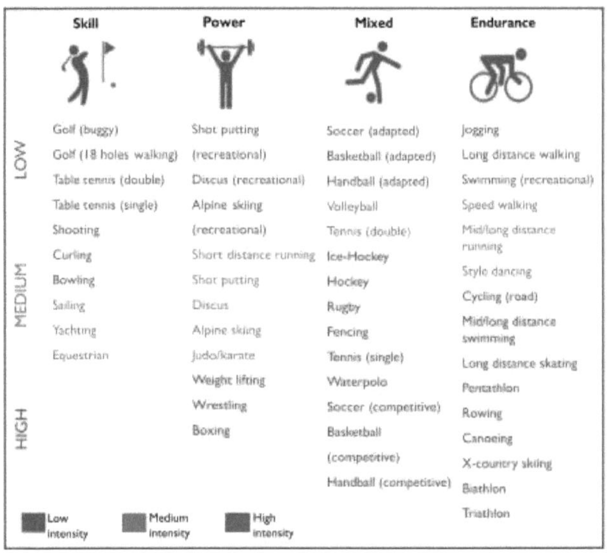

Figure 1: Classification of sports according to the predominant component (skill, power, mixed or endurance) and intensity of exercise. According to the ESC 2020 Guidelines on Sports Cardiology (20).

III.   RISK OF SPORTS-RELATED INJURY

The National Hemophilia Foundation (NHF) published a patient document in 2017 entitled "Playing it Safe-Bleeding Disorders, Sports and Exercise," in which it provides a comprehensive list of sports with associated risk of injury (21).

Each sport is rated according to four levels of risk: low (1), low to moderate (1.5), moderate (2), moderate to high (2.5) and high (3). The risk levels have been created using population injury statistics and can be used as a resource for doctors and patients.

Table 1 summarises common sports and their associated risk levels.

Table I: Risk levels

NHF risk levels	1-1,5	1,5-2	2-2,5	3
Sports	- Water exercise - Archery - Flying disc - Golf - Rowing - Freediving - Swimming - Tai chi - Tee-ball	- Bowling - Recreational diving - Flag / Touch Football - Indoor climbing - Running / jogging - Cross-country skiing - Tennis - Yoga	- Baseball - Basketball - Cycling - Cheerleading - Riding - Mountain biking - Underwater diving - Skateboarding - Ice skating - Downhill skiing - Water skiing -Softball - Surfing - Athletics - Racquetball - Volleyball	- BMX race - Boxing - Competition diving -Gymnastics - Hockey - Martial arts - Motorbikes / motocross - The stick - Power lifting - Rodeo - Rugby - Snowmobile - Football - Trampoline - Fighting

IV. ADVERSE CARDIOVASCULAR EVENTS
MAJOR EVENTS RELATING TO THE FINANCIAL YEAR

Higher levels of physical activity are associated with lower all-cause mortality, lower rates of cardiovascular disease and a lower prevalence of several known malignancies (22-30).

Despite the substantial health benefits provided by regular physical activity, intense exercise can paradoxically act as a trigger for potentially fatal ventricular arrhythmias in the presence of underlying cardiovascular disease.

Major exercise-related cardiovascular adverse events include cardiac arrest and sudden death; acute coronary syndromes such as myocardial ischaemia and myocardial infarction; transient ischaemic attack and stroke; and supraventricular tachyarrhythmias.

V. MAIN PATHOLOGIES REQUIRING ANTICOAGULANT TREATMENT IN ATHLETES

<u>AF</u> and <u>thromboembolic venous disease</u> are the main pathologies affecting sportsmen and women that may require anticoagulant treatment.

According to recent estimates, the prevalence of AF is around 3% in adults aged 20 or over (31) and increases with age (32).

The estimated incidence of DVT is around 1 per 1,000 adults (33), a number that is probably underestimated because many cases of asymptomatic DVT may be misdiagnosed.

Other less frequent indications for anticoagulation in sportsmen and women include pulmonary embolism and previous valve implantation.

V.1 SUPRAVENTRICULAR ARRHYTHMIAS

V.1.1 ATRIAL FIBRILLATION IN ATHLETES

The expression "mhdén ágan" is engraved in the temple of Apollo at Delphi.

This ancient Greek proverb - "nothing in excess" - characterises the belief that a healthy life is achieved by following the principle of moderation.

Atrial fibrillation (AF) in the high-intensity endurance athlete highlights the concept that even healthy behaviours can have harmful effects when performed in excess.

Although athletes with AF represent a small subset of all patients with this common arrhythmia, this sporting population intrigues the medical community and the public.

Historically and in contemporary culture, athletes are symbols of health.

Exercise as the driving force behind the pathophysiology of arrhythmia therefore appears to contradict the known cardiovascular benefits of physical activity.

V.1.1.1 -Epidemiology

Several case-control studies and retrospective analyses first demonstrated a higher prevalence of AF associated with long-term vigorous training (34,35).

Additional studies and subsequent meta-analyses have supported these results (36-41).

On the basis of these data, the frequency of AF was estimated to be 2 to 10 times higher in high-intensity endurance athletes than in sedentary individuals.

However, most of this evidence has the limitation of being retrospective and observational. What's more, most of this data has been collected from relatively small populations of athletes.

In an American registry including 16,921 healthy men (42), vigorous exercise was associated with an increased risk of developing AF in young men (under 50) and joggers.

Compared to men who did not exercise vigorously, men who jogged 5 to 7 times a week had a risk of
significantly increased risk of developing AF (relative risk [RR]:
1.53, 95% confidence interval [CI]: 1.12 to 2.09; p<0.01).

The frequency of cardiac arrhythmias was also assessed in more than 52,000 competitive cross-country skiers in Sweden (43). AF occurred in 681 skiers (HR: 13.2; 95% CI: 12.3 to 14.3 / 10,000 person-years at risk). The frequency of AF in this cohort increased in proportion to the number of 90 km races completed (HR: 1.29; 95% CI: 1.04 to 1.61 for 5 races completed vs 1 race completed).

These observations were also supported by a Norwegian longitudinal study of 162,078 women and 147,462 men (44). The
The investigators found that 575 men (0.4%) and 288 women (0.2%) were classified as having AF. The risk of AF increased with self-reported levels of physical activity.

In a meta-analysis of six case-control studies, Nielsen et al. showed that the risk of AF increased > 5 times in athletes compared with non-athletic controls (OR: 5.3; 95% CI: 3.6 to 7.9; p <0.0001) (45). Moderate or high intensity of usual physical activity was associated with a significantly reduced risk of AF compared with low intensity or no physical activity (OR: 0.89; 95% CI: 0.83 to 0.96; p <0.0001) (28). The authors thus concluded that long-term vigorous physical training or a lack of physical activity were both associated with an increased risk of AF. In contrast, habitual moderate physical activity was associated with a reduced risk (45).

On the basis of individual studies and meta-analyses, the concept of a "J" model describing the relationship between exercise and AF has been put forward (39,40,42,44- 47) (Figure 2). Thus, regular exercise of mild to moderate intensity offers protection against cardiovascular disease and AF, while more sustained endurance exercise may increase the burden of AF.

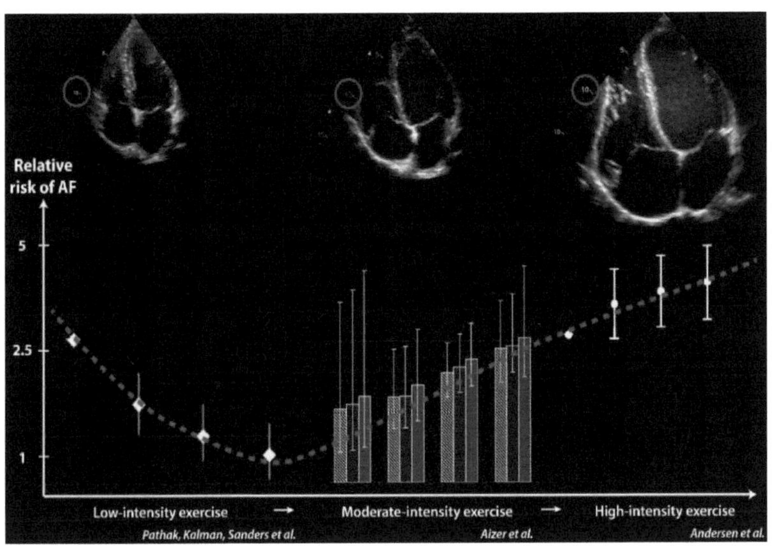

Figure 2: J-shaped relationship between exercise dose and relative risk of developing AF. Echocardiograms are shown in relative scale demonstrating the increase in heart and atrial size with exercise. Adapted from La Gerche et al. Eur Heart J 2013.

Much of the reported data on exercise and AF has been largely focused on males. A recent meta-analysis of the relationship between AF and exercise suggests that there may be a sex-specific effect.

(48). Although moderate physical activity was protective in men (OR: 0.81; 95% CI: 0.26 to 1.004; p = 0.06), vigorous physical activity was associated with a significantly increased risk of AF (OR: 3.30; 95% CI: 1.97 to 4.63; p = 0.0002) (48). In contrast, pooled analysis of data from 149,048 women showed that those involved in moderate physical activity had an 8.6% lower risk of developing AF (OR: 0.91; 95% CI: 0.77 to 0.97; p = 0.002), intense exercise was even more protective, conferring a 28% lower risk of AF compared with sedentary control subjects (OR: 0.72; 95% CI: 0.57 to 0.88; p <0.001) (48) (Figure 3).

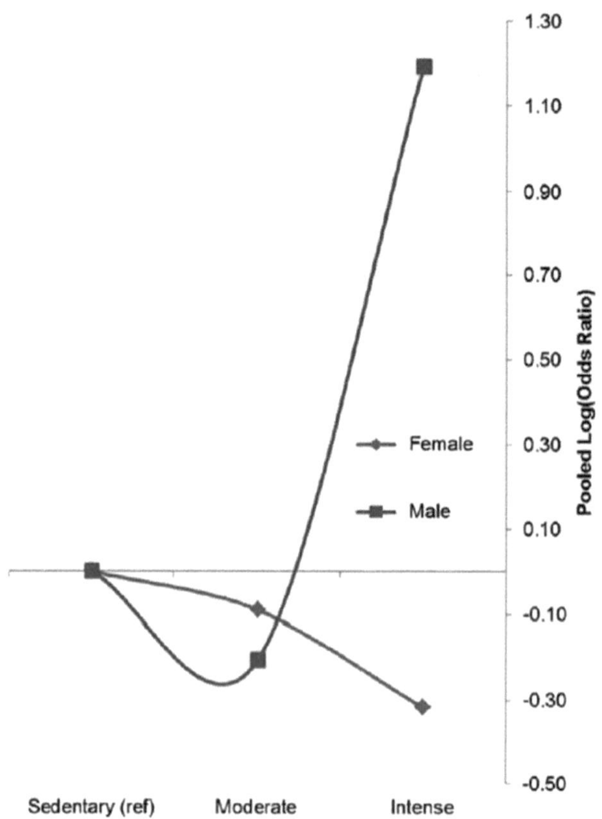

Figure 3: Association between level of physical activity and risk of AF according to sex (48).

V.1.1.2 -Pathophysiology

There are many gaps in our knowledge of the pathophysiological mechanisms that promote the development of AF in athletes.

Proposed mechanisms include alterations in autonomic tone, left atrial dilatation and fibrosis, electrical remodelling and increased inflammation (49-53).

Although these mechanisms are complex and are likely to vary between individuals, there is consensus that common elements include autonomic, structural and electro-physiological remodelling that predisposes to triggered activity from the pulmonary veins or re-entry into atrial tissue (49-53) (Figure 3).

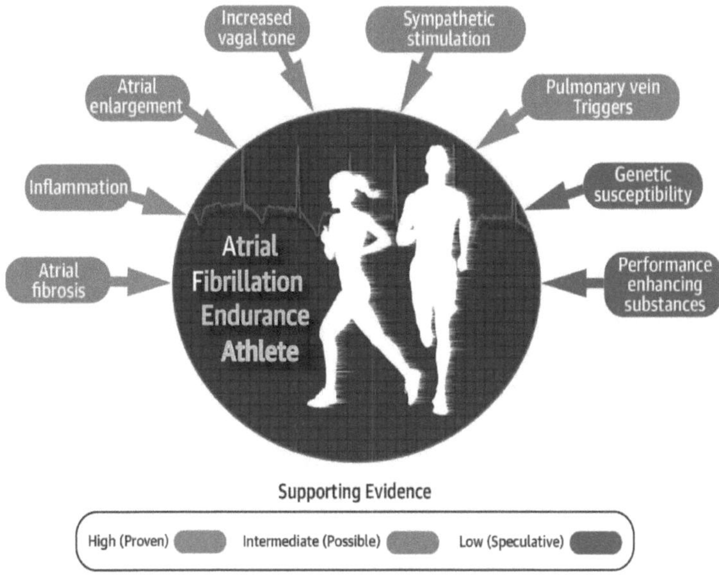

Figure 4: Pathophysiological mechanisms of AF in endurance athletes. Adapted from Estes and Madias (54).

Clinical studies have shown that at rest and during low-intensity physical activity, endurance athletes have a predominant vagal tone compared with non-athletes (51,55,56).

Increased vagal activity is known to shorten the atrial refractory period through activation of the iKAch channel (49-53).

It has been postulated that a wave-induced decrease in the refractory period and a slowed atrial conduction velocity may facilitate reentry. Alterations in autonomic tone, including an exercise-related intermittent increase in sympathetic tone in endurance athletes, may also predispose to AF (57-61). In many athletes, AF occurs at night when vagal tone is more pronounced (59). In these individuals, sinus bradycardia and atrioventricular block are frequently observed during sleep (59,60).

In conclusion, it is well recognised that the development of AF, like other arrhythmias, depends on several factors: triggers, substrates and modulators.

Atrial extrasystoles, particularly near the pulmonary veins, have been indicated as a trigger in most episodes of AF.

As far as the substrate is concerned, structural remodelling and fibrosis of the left atrium is a major risk factor for the development of AF.

Vagal tone could be a key modulator of AF in athletes.

Genetic factors may also play a role in the development of AF.

Finally, another factor to consider when investigating AF in athletes is the potential use of illicit substances. The use of anabolic steroids has been suggested as a potential cause of AF.

V.1.1.3 -Diagnosis of atrial fibrillation in athletes

Athletes with palpitations require careful assessment.

Initial assessment includes a physical examination and a 12-lead electrocardiogram (ECG). However, paroxysmal AF is often missed on the standard ECG despite a suggestive clinical history.

Prolonged ECG monitoring is recommended for any suspected but undocumented episode of AF.

In non-athletes, it has been estimated that a 7-day Holter ECG recording can document the arrhythmia in around 70% of affected patients. For the moment, there are no data concerning more prolonged monitoring with an implantable holter, and according to the guidelines, apart from certain cases, these devices should be considered for documenting AF in stroke patients (62).

The ECG may also indicate the presence of other underlying cardiovascular conditions (e.g. cardiomyopathy, coronary artery disease) associated with AF.

Analysis of the P-wave signal is rarely used in clinical practice: however, a duration greater than 145 ms predicts the transition from paroxysmal to persistent AF. In athletes, mean P-wave duration can help differentiate vagal AF from AF secondary to atrial remodelling (36).

In addition, echocardiography and laboratory tests should be carried out to rule out common causes of AF, such as structural heart disease, electrolyte disorders or thyroid dysfunction.

V.1.1.4 -Indications for anticoagulant treatment of AF in athletes
In the case of AF, the indication for long-term anticoagulation depends on the thromboembolic risk determined according to scores such as the CHADS2 or CHA2DS2-VASc score (62). This is the score most commonly used in clinical practice. It is determined by assigning one or two points to the following parameters: congestive heart failure, hypertension, age ≥ 75 years (2 points), diabetes, stroke (2 points), vascular disease, age 65 to 74 years and female sex (63).

Anticoagulation to prevent thromboembolic events due to AF is recommended in all male patients with a CHA2DS2-VASc score of 2 or more and in all female patients with a score of 3 or more (Class I, Level A) (64). Anticoagulation should also be considered for men with a CHA2DS2-VASc score of 1 and women with a score of 2, taking into account several aspects such as expected stroke reduction, bleeding risk and patient preference.

Thus, patients under 65 with no other thromboembolic risk factors have no indication for anticoagulation, unless they are undergoing pharmacological or electrical cardioversion or catheter ablation, in which case anticoagulation for 4 weeks is recommended to avoid the risk of stroke associated with so-called "atrial stunning" (65). Some of these subjects (under 65 years of age with an indication for temporary anticoagulation treatment) probably take part in competitive sports, which raises the question of whether and how physical activity can be authorised during anticoagulation.

Furthermore, with regard to AF ablation, it should be considered that after the ablative procedure, each subject should continue anticoagulation for a period, generally for at least three months. After this period, the decision to stop anticoagulation should be based on the VASc CHA2DS2 score, independently of the ablative results.

V.1.2 ATRIAL FLUTTER

Many series report the presence of both AF and flutter in endurance athletes.

Hoogsteen et al (66) found that atrial flutter was present in 10% of athletes with paroxysmal AF.

Baldesberger et al (67) evaluated arrhythmias in long-term follow-up (30 to 50 years) after high-endurance training in former professional cyclists, and found that atrial flutter was more frequent than AF.

Heidbuchel et al (68) described a higher incidence of AF after flutter ablation in endurance athletes than in controls. According to these authors, flutter ablation could unmask underlying atrial disease in endurance athletes, leading to the development of AF during follow-up.

On the basis of these results, endurance sport may contribute to the development of both arrhythmias.

V.2 THROMBOEMBOLIC VENOUS DISEASE

Venous thromboembolism (VTE) in professional athletes is a serious condition, often requiring long-term anticoagulant treatment with life- or career-threatening consequences. VTE is a term that encompasses deep vein thrombosis (DVT) of the upper limbs, DVT of the lower limbs and pulmonary embolism (PE).

V.2.1 DEEP VEIN THROMBOSIS

V.2.1.1 -Epidemiology

The occurrence of venous thrombosis in sportsmen and women remains rare. Between 0.5% and 2.5% per year (OR 0.7%) of venous thrombotic events are reported for every 1,000 subjects practising more than one hour of sport per week (the figures are higher for sedentary people) (69). This variation is linked to age, with the risk of thrombosis increasing threefold over the age of 60. The intensity at which sport is practised is not a factor in triggering venous accidents, which are more often associated with endurance than resistance sports (69).

In the general population, the majority of DVTs occur in the lower limbs. Upper limb DVT is rare, occurring in approximately 2 per 100,000 people per year, but it is the most common vascular condition in athletes (70). Bishop et al (71) report the rate of isolated lower limb DVT as 27% of total thromboembolic events in a sports population.

V.2.1.2 -Pathophysiology

The development of thrombosis is summarised by Virchow's triad of endothelial damage, blood stasis and blood hyperviscosity (Figure 5). These three factors predisposing to clot formation trigger a cascade of procoagulant reactions culminating in thrombus formation.

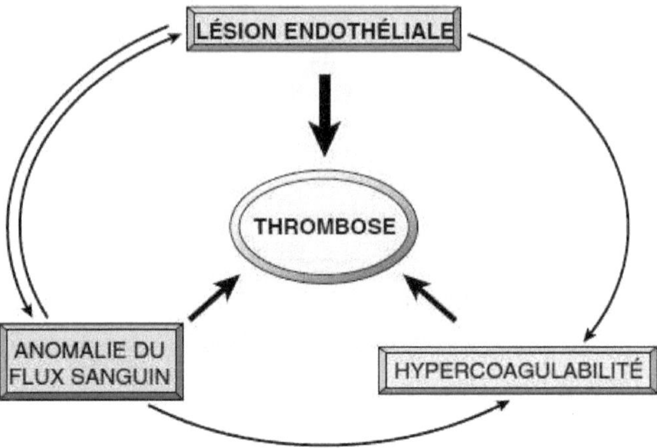

Figure 5: Virchow triad

> ➤ DVT of the lower limbs :

DVT is most often associated with venous stasis in the deep veins of the calf or pelvis, with the incidence increasing with age.

Risk factors such as trauma, surgery and immobilisation all contribute to thrombus formation, which depends on Virchow's triad.

Exercise has been shown to disrupt homeostatic mechanisms (72). The degree of disruption depends on the intensity of the exercise, with high-intensity training increasing both prothrombotic and fibrinolytic markers. (73). There are no specific sports known to predispose to this condition. However, it appears that any activity involving trauma to the lower limbs, either blunt trauma or repetitive strain, increases the risk of developing thrombosis.

The pathological mechanisms favouring athlete-specific DVT are multifactorial.

In endurance athletes, venous compression by surrounding structures can cause microtrauma, endothelial cell damage and subsequent activation of the coagulation cascade (74). Blunt trauma, especially in contact sports, may also predispose these individuals to DVT of the lower limbs. Other physiological factors contributing to a prothrombotic environment specific to this patient population include dehydration, increased flight time due to travel and bradycardia leading to venous stasis (71,75,76).

Idiopathic thrombus formation in athletes is rare, but should be suspected in low-risk individuals with oedematous, erythematous and painful limbs (74).

In young, active patients, it is important to exclude underlying conditions predisposing to venous thrombosis, including thrombophilias such as factor V Leiden and protein C deficiency, as their presence increases recurrence rates.

> ➤ DVT of the upper limbs

Between 4% and 10% of all DVT events in the general population involve the upper limb (77).

Primary DVT of the upper limbs is idiopathic in nature and accounts for 20% of cases of upper limb DVT (78).

Secondary DVT of the upper limbs most commonly occurs as a result of systemic disease or venous catheterisation (79). Complications include symptomatic PE, post-thrombotic syndrome and recurrence after treatment (77). The risk of PE varies between 2% and 36% of cases of upper limb DVT (77) and appears to be less frequent than in the case of lower limb DVT.

According to a study of injury reports from the National Hockey League, Major League Baseball, the National Basketball Association and the National Football League in the United States, collating only active professional athletes, upper limb DVT was particularly prevalent in baseball players (68.9% of reported cases) compared with the other groups, highlighting their increased risk associated with the repetitive upper limb movements that these athletes perform (71).

A subgroup of primary DVT of the upper limbs is known as <u>Paget-Schroetter syndrome</u> (exertional thrombosis).

It is part of the thoracic outlet syndrome, a group of disorders manifested by vascular or neurological symptoms of the upper limbs secondary to compression of the neurovascular structures in the thoracic outlet.

Although rare, with an incidence of 1 to 2 per 100,000 people per year (80), it is an important complication in athletes performing extensive upper-limb exercise, including baseball players, swimmers and wrestlers (81).

Although the exact aetiology remains unknown, the presence of scar tissue surrounding the vasculature observed intraoperatively in these individuals suggests a chronic inflammatory process secondary to repetitive trauma of arm abduction and external rotation. Thrombosis probably occurs at a later stage after platelet activation and deposition. A number of other factors, including muscle hypertrophy, have also been implicated in the pathology of exercise-induced thrombosis (82).

V.2.1.3 -Diagnosis of DVT in athletes
The diagnosis of DVT in athletes follows the same pattern as in the general population. The presenting symptoms of DVT include symmetrical swelling of the extremities, erythema and oedema.

When assessing an athlete, clinicians need to be vigilant about the risk of misdiagnosing DVT. For example, symptoms due to DVT may be wrongly attributed to a muscle strain or tear (83). Athletes' potential unwillingness to disclose symptoms of the disease, their baseline bradycardia and higher pain threshold may not attract the clinician's attention for further investigation.

Venous ultrasound is recommended for the diagnosis of DVT (84). When the clinical suspicion of DVT is high and ultrasound is negative, angioscan or magnetic resonance imaging may be used.

V.2.1.4   -Indications for anticoagulant treatment in DVT

In the case of DVT, three months' curative anticoagulation is indicated (85).

In cases of unprovoked proximal DVT or pulmonary embolism with permanent thrombotic risk factors, long-term anticoagulation should be considered (86).

V.2.2 PULMONARY EMBOLISM

PE is rare in athletes, particularly in the younger population, and few cases have been reported (74,87,88).

As a result, PE is often under-reported among athletes.

There are many risk factors for the development of PE, including hereditary conditions, immobilisation, recent surgery, stroke, a history of thromboembolism, advanced age and neoplasia. Although these factors are not often observed in the sporting population, the use of oral contraceptives is widespread. Oral contraceptives cause a slight but significant increase in the risk of thromboembolic events associated with the duration of use and the type of contraceptive.

The clinical diagnosis of PE is difficult. Patients present with variable symptoms such as dyspnoea, pleuritic pain, cough and haemoptysis. The most common presenting sign is tachypnoea, but may also include tachycardia, hypoxaemia or fever.

As in the general population, the Wells criteria can guide the pre-test probability of PE, and CT pulmonary angiography is the gold standard.

V.2.3 SUPERFICIAL VENOUS THROMBOSIS

Superficial thrombophlebitis (SST) is thought to occur more frequently than DVT, but is not as well studied (89).

There is limited evidence to guide the choice and duration of treatment if anticoagulation is indicated.

The American College of CHEST physicians recommends treating DVT of the lower limbs with prophylactic doses of fondaparinux or low molecular weight heparin for 45 days (89).

Similarly, Di Nisio et al (90) recommend a prophylactic dose of fondaparinux for 6 weeks.

However, Hill et al (91) argue that proximal great saphenous vein DVT should be treated in the same way as lower limb DVT because it may be associated with a similar mortality rate.

Close monitoring by venous ultrasound is necessary to ensure that the thrombus does not spread. In addition, compression stockings are recognised as a mainstay of treatment.

VI.   ANTICOAGULANTS

Anticoagulant therapy can be administered orally or parenterally. The latter is not suitable for long-term use and is generally administered in hospital as an overlap therapy to oral therapy. It involves heparin, low molecular weight heparins and heparinoids such as fondaparinux.

VI.1 CHARACTERISTICS OF ORAL ANTICOAGULANTS

Although anti-vitamin K (AVK) agents (warfarin and acenocumarol) were for years a cornerstone of oral anticoagulation (92), they are now generally reserved for cases where direct oral anticoagulants (AOD) are contraindicated, such as the presence of a valve prosthesis, valvular atrial fibrillation, intra-ventricular thrombus and in general in all cases where AODs are contraindicated by the technical data sheet.

VKAs are antagonists of vitamin K-dependent hepatic proteins and reduce circulating levels of factors II, VII, IX and X. This pharmacodynamic property requires 3-5 days to achieve a complete anticoagulant effect (INR>2), necessitating overlapping treatment with a parenteral anticoagulant (93). Given this pharmacodynamic property, VKAs are also very slow to be eliminated (93).

AODs were designed to overcome the limitations of VKAs, which include delayed action and elimination, a narrow therapeutic interval, several drug and food interactions, a variable and unpredictable effect, the influence of CYP2A9 and VKORC1 genetic polymorphism, a labile INR and the need for frequent monitoring (93,94).

There are currently four AODs: dabigatran, apixaban, rivaroxaban and edoxaban (95). Only the first is a prodrug and selectively inhibits thrombin; the others are selective inhibitors of activated factor X. All AODs are reversible enzyme inhibitors.

Their bioavailability is influenced in various ways by concomitant food intake.

After absorption, AODs reach peak plasma levels in approximately 2 to 3 hours. They have a half-life of around 12 hours and elimination is mainly renal for dabigatran and hepatic and renal for apixaban, rivaroxaban and edoxaban (96). For this reason, it is important to take into account renal function, as well as other demographic characteristics, to establish the most appropriate AOD and the correct dosage for each patient (96).
Dabigatran, apixaban and edoxaban are contraindicated in patients with severe hepatic impairment (Child-Pugh C), while rivaroxaban is also contraindicated in patients with moderate hepatic impairment (Child-Pugh B).

Dabigatran and apixaban should be taken twice daily, while rivaroxaban and edoxaban once daily. Furthermore, elimination of the drugs may vary according to the AOD and their residual activity may not be negligible even 24 hours after the last dose, as reported by Sairaku et al (97).

This aspect should be borne in mind when choosing anticoagulant therapy for sportsmen and women.

Table II summarises the pharmacokinetic and pharmacodynamic characteristics of warfarin and the various ODAs.

Table II: Main characteristics of warfarin and AODs

	Warfarin	Dabigatran	Apixaban	Edoxaban	Rivaroxaban
Target	Factors II, VII, IX and X	Thrombin	Xa	Xa	Xa
Prodrug	No	Yes	No	No	No
Reversibility of inhibition	No	Yes	Yes	Yes	Yes
Bioavailability	100%	3-7%	50%	62%	66% (80-100% with food)
Effect of the plug food	No	Delayed	No	No	Increased
Volume of distribution (L)	10	60-70	21	>300	50
Link plas. proteins	99%	35%	87%	40-59%	>90%
Concentration maximum (H)	2-4	1-3	3-4	2	2-4
Half-life (H)	40	12-17	12	10-14	5-9
Elimination kidney	0%	80%	27%	35%	33%
Purification by HD	No	60-70%	Little probable	Possible	Unlikely
Number of sockets / J	1	2	2	1	1
Shape galenic	Tablet	Capsule	Tablet	Tablet	Tablet

Table III summarises the clinical indications and doses of AODs.

Table III: Indications and doses of AODs

	Prevention of TE in non-valvular AF	Curative treatment of DVT and PE	Prevention of recurrence of DVT and PE	Prevention of TE after orthopaedic surgery	Primary prevention after ACS without AF	Secondary prevention in heart disease Ischaemic and arterial disease peripheral
Dabigatran	150 mg*2/d or 110 mg*2/ d If : • ≥80 years or • verapamil	Start with parenteral anticoagulation for 5 days, then 150 mg (or 110 mg if of age) >80 years or verapamil)*2/d	150 mg*2/d or 110 mg*2 /d If : • ≥80 years or • verapamil	220 mg/d or 150 mg/d if : • ≥80 years or • verapamil	-	-
Apixaban	5 mg*2/d or 2.5 mg*2/d if : ≥80 years, ≤ 60 kg, serum creatinine ≥ 1.5 mg/dl (133 µmol/l)	10 mg*2/d for 7 days then 5 mg*2/d (3 months)	2.5 mg*2/d	2.5 mg*2/d	-	-
	60 mg/d or 30 mg/d if :	Start with anticoag. Parenteral :				

Edoxaban	≤ 60 kg, ClCr <50 mL/min, verapamil or quinidine	for 5 days then 60 mg/d or 30 mg/d if: ≤ 60 kg, CrCl <50 mL/min, verapamil or quinidine	No scientific proof	Not approved in Europe	-	-
Rivaroxaban	20 mg/d or 15 mg/d if ClCr <50 mL/min	15 mg *2/d for 21 days then 20 mg/d	10 mg/d or 20 mg/d if high risk	10 mg/d	2.5 mg*2/d + Asp + inh P2Y12 (ATLAS ACS 2-TIMI 51) (98)	2.5 mg*2d +Asp (COMPASS) (99)

VI.2 CONDUCT IN THE EVENT OF BLEEDING UNDER AOD

In the event of haemorrhage on an AOD, the course of action varies according to the severity of the haemorrhage.

In the event of minor bleeding, simply delay or temporarily suspend the use of the drug in combination with local haemostatic and/or aetiological treatment.

In the event of recurrent haemorrhage, it may be useful to change the AOD.

In the event of major haemorrhage that is not life-threatening, in addition to the above measures, activated charcoal (if AOD has recently been taken), blood derivatives, haemodynamic support, platelet concentrates if plq<60000, desmopressin (if coagulopathy present), tranexamic acid (1 g every 6 hours) should be considered.

For haemorrhages on dabigatran, the administration of the specific antidote idarucizumab (5 mg IV in two doses 15 minutes apart) should be considered, or haemodialysis should be envisaged, bearing in mind that this is effective in the first few hours following administration, given the drug's high volume of distribution.

All of the above strategies should be implemented in the event of life-threatening bleeding in association with the administration of idarucizumab with or without prothrombin complex (PPSB) if dabigatran is used, or only PPSB if anti-Xa is used (93).

Andexanet alfa was approved in 2018 by the FDA and in 2019 by the European Medicines Agency (EMA) as an antidote to apixaban and rivaroxaban. However, trials on this drug are still ongoing (93).

VII.   SPORT AND ANTICOAGULANTS :

VII.1-What do the recommendations say?

The major risk for athletes on anticoagulant therapy arises from potential 'body-to-body' or 'object-to-body' impacts occurring during training or competition, as these increase the risk of serious injury, particularly intracranial haemorrhage.

For some sports, impact is inevitable, such as football, volleyball and hockey. For other sports, impact is unlikely, such as golf, running and swimming.

The recommendations of **the 36th Bethesda Conference** state that AF patients on long-term anticoagulation should not take part in sports involving the risk of body contact or the danger of trauma (100), as also emphasised **in the European recommendations for the practice of recreational and competitive sports in patients with arrhythmias and potentially arrhythmogenic conditions** (68).

The consensus of the **ESC Sports Cardiology Study Group** recommends only mild to moderate static or dynamic activities, and prohibits all contact sports for athletes on anticoagulation (7).

The AHA / ACC consensus (101) recommends that :

• athletes taking VKAs or OADs should not participate in impact sports due to the increased risk of intracranial haemorrhage (class III, level of evidence C)

• athletes with a history of AF and on long-term anticoagulation should not participate in sports involving the risk of body contact (class III, level of evidence C)

• Athletes with mechanical aortic or mitral valve prostheses on anticoagulants with normal LV function can reasonably participate in low-intensity competitive sports if there is a low probability of body contact (Class IIa; Level of Evidence C).

The Italian Sports Cardiology Committee (COCIS) (102) states that permanent AF generally contraindicates eligibility for competitive sport requiring moderate to high cardiovascular demand. Eligibility can only be granted for skill sports (pétanque, bowling, curling, skittles, golf, fishing, shooting sports, sport hunting, billiards, bridge, draughts, chess) and when the sporting activity does not involve a high risk of trauma for people on anticoagulants.

VII.2 What does the literature say?

There are few data in the literature on anticoagulation and sporting activity, mainly consisting of case reports, mostly relating to warfarin treatment.

In recent years, attention to anticoagulation and sport has increased since the introduction of OADs into clinical practice. Some recent articles provide suggestions for trying to implement a new approach to anticoagulation management in athletes.

Berkowitz et al (103), with reference to the treatment of DVT, suggest that the risk of bleeding in an athlete on an AOD can be minimised with a pharmacokinetic and pharmacodynamic study in which the athlete ingests the AOD and repeated measurements of the plasma concentration of the drug are taken over 24 hours. By obtaining several plasma concentrations of the drug over this period, a determination of the elimination half-life of the drug can be made and the level of plasma concentration of the drug correlated with the minimal risk of bleeding can be identified. In this way, the intake of the AOD can be programmed so that its plasma level has reached a level below the threshold correlated with an increased risk of bleeding at the time of sports practice. At the end of the sporting event, when the risk of trauma or haemorrhage has returned to normal, a dose of the drug can be taken, with a rapid onset of the anticoagulant effect.

Given the inter- and intra-individual fluctuations in the plasma concentration of AODs, particularly dabigatran (104-106), it is important to carry out an individualised study by taking several blood samples during the day, simulating the athlete's competition schedule if possible, and then repeating the study to confirm the data initially determined.

Moll et al (105) consider a residual level of rivaroxaban and apixaban of less than 30 ng/mL to be potentially safe for the athlete engaged in collision and contact activities. In addition, they propose a strategy of intermittent use of AOD in the long-term management of athletes with a history of DVT allowing them to return to full sporting activity by stopping the drug some time before sporting activities considered at risk of bleeding and restarting it immediately afterwards if no significant trauma has occurred.

Sanna et al (107) argue that AODs should be preferred in athletes with AF and an indication for anticoagulation, due to their advantages (no INR monitoring, minor drug and food interactions, etc.) which improve compliance in this group of patients. In addition, they address a controversial issue which is the decision to anticoagulate athletes with a CHA2DS2-VASc score of 1 (apart from gender), which is the most common condition encountered in sports populations, due to the low cardiovascular risk profile (as often only hypertension is present). On this subject, there is a major discrepancy between the recommendations of the ESC and the AHA/ACC. The ESC gives anticoagulation in these subjects a class IIa recommendation, level of evidence B (62), whereas the AHA (108) suggests the possibility of therapeutic abstention, using aspirin or anticoagulants in this case. Sanna et al. support the European approach, arguing that the score does not include other possible risk factors leading to a high thromboembolic risk (such as renal failure, obstructive sleep apnoea, etc.) and suggest that anticoagulation with AOD should be carefully considered in athletes with AF and a CHA2DS2-VASc score of 1 apart from gender.

VII.3 What can we learn from the guidelines and the literature?

Non-contact sports, such as running and swimming, are characterised by a low probability of trauma.

Sports such as baseball and volleyball are defined as *limited-contact sports* because contact is involuntary and infrequent.

Contact sports are those in which some degree of trauma occurs regularly during play, such as basketball and football.

Collision sports, such as American football and ice hockey, involve a great deal of body contact.

Although participation in non-contact sports is considered safe without interruption of anticoagulant therapy, all international recommendations (7,20,100-102,109) agree that participation in limited-contact, contact and collision sports is not recommended.

However, the majority of recommendations derive from the management of anticoagulants before the introduction of AODs into clinical practice. Given their pharmacokinetic and pharmacodynamic properties, AODs are a promising resource for continuing physical activity without stopping anticoagulant treatment.

An individualised approach could be proposed. To achieve this, a distinction must first be made between cases in which anticoagulation is indicated for the treatment of an existing thromboembolic disease (such as DVT, PE, thrombus in the left atrium) and cases in which it is used to prevent thromboembolic events.

In the first case, any sporting activity that increases the risk of haemorrhage should be avoided, as it is absolutely incompatible with stopping anticoagulant treatment, given the high risk of embolisms.

In the case of prophylaxis, the AOD could offer the possibility of implementing a sort of "therapeutic window" scheme (104,105) outside which, when the anticoagulant effect is complete or minimal, sporting activity involving a variable degree of contact can be carried out safely.

While intermittent use of AOD for prophylaxis may be safer in subjects who engage in leisure-time physical activity with occasional exercise sessions, it is less suitable for athletes who train regularly (2-3 times a week), and even less safe for those who exercise daily.

These strategies could perhaps represent a solution for elite athletes, for whom suspension of physical activity has greater economic and psychological implications.

In this context, AODs with short half-lives or those administered twice daily may be useful. Of course, the availability of an antidote that rapidly reverses the anticoagulant effects may represent an additional advantage and a selection criterion.

When sporting activity has taken place without traumatic events, anticoagulant treatment can reasonably be resumed within 1 to 2 hours. In the case of trauma, a much longer delay for resumption of treatment is suggested as a safer option (104).

It should also be pointed out that there is insufficient evidence to support the use of left atrial closure in athletes, and further studies should be carried out to determine its therapeutic usefulness.

Finally, there remains the problem of who should authorise sporting activity in the presence of anticoagulant treatment, even with regimes which provide for discontinuous intake. Given that this is not authorised by the guidelines and that there is currently insufficient evidence and studies to support such conduct, the cardiologist or sports doctor who advises him or her could be exposed to medico-legal problems in the event of haemorrhage or thromboembolic events.

CONCLUSIONS

Physical activity has both preventive and therapeutic benefits. Consequently, prohibiting all subjects on anticoagulants from practising sport because of their increased risk of bleeding could be disadvantageous.

The optimal management of anticoagulation in sports professionals and ordinary people practising physical activity is unclear, and solid evidence is lacking.

Physical activities with a low risk of trauma should be recommended, even in patients on anticoagulants, as a preventive strategy, and the use of AODs can make the possibility of trauma, which should however be limited, more manageable.

In addition, the pharmacological profile of the new oral anticoagulants already offers theoretical solutions to the increased risk of haemorrhage in this category of patients. For example, the choice of drugs with a shorter half-life may be a solution for patients who sporadically take part in sports with a high risk of trauma.

Further studies are needed to find out how anticoagulant therapy can be appropriately managed in athletes to minimise the risk of bleeding and enable them to pursue their careers safely, probably by means of an individual clinical assessment, taking into account all the risks and benefits associated with taking part or not taking part in a sporting activity, as well as the type of sport and anticoagulant therapy, and also involving patient-athletes in clinical decision-making.

REFERENCES

1. 2018 Physical Activity Guidelines Advisory Committee Scientific Report. :779.

2. Piepoli MF, Hoes AW, Agewall S, Albus C, Brotons C, Catapano AL, et al. 2016 European Guidelines on cardiovascular disease prevention in clinical practiceThe Sixth Joint Task Force of the European Society of Cardiology and Other Societies on Cardiovascular Disease Prevention in Clinical Practice (constituted by representatives of 10 societies and by invited experts)Developed with the special contribution of the European Association for Cardiovascular Prevention & Rehabilitation (EACPR). Eur Heart J. 1 August 2016;37(29):2315-81.

3. Lee I-M, Shiroma EJ, Lobelo F, Puska P, Blair SN, Katzmarzyk PT, et al. Effect of physical inactivity on major non-communicable diseases worldwide: an analysis of burden of disease and life expectancy. Lancet. 21 Jul 2012;380(9838):219-29.

4. Giannuzzi P, Temporelli PL, Marchioli R, Maggioni AP, Balestroni G, Ceci V, et al. Global secondary prevention strategies to limit event recurrence after myocardial infarction: results of the GOSPEL study, a multicenter, randomized controlled trial from the Italian Cardiac Rehabilitation Network. Arch Intern Med. 10 Nov 2008;168(20):2194-204.

5. Mezzani A, Hamm LF, Jones AM, McBride PE, Moholdt T, Stone JA, et al. Aerobic exercise intensity assessment and prescription in cardiac rehabilitation: A joint position statement of the European Association for Cardiovascular Prevention and Rehabilitation, the American Association of Cardiovascular and Pulmonary Rehabilitation and the Canadian Association of Cardiac Rehabilitation. European journal of preventive cardiology. 2013;20(3):442-67.

6. Solberg Ee, Borjesson M, Sharma S, Papadakis M, Wilhelm M, Drezner Ja, et al. Sudden cardiac arrest in sports - need for uniform registration: A Position Paper from the Sport Cardiology Section of the European Association for Cardiovascular Prevention and Rehabilitation [Internet]. Vol. 23, European journal of preventive cardiology. Eur J Prev Cardiol; 2016 [cited 23 Oct 2020]. Available from: https://pubmed.ncbi.nlm.nih.gov/26285770/

7. Pelliccia A, Fagard R, Bjørnstad Hh, Anastassakis A, Arbustini E, Assanelli D, et al. Recommendations for competitive sports participation in athletes with cardiovascular disease: a consensus document from the Study Group of Sports Cardiology of the Working Group of Cardiac Rehabilitation and Exercise Physiology and the Working Group of Myocardial and Pericardial Diseases of the European Society of Cardiology [Internet]. Vol. 26, European heart journal. Eur Heart J; 2005 [cited 23 Oct 2020]. Available from: https://pubmed.ncbi.nlm.nih.gov/15923204/

8. Drezner Ja, Peterson Df, Siebert Dm, Thomas Lc, Lopez-Anderson M, Suchsland Mz, et al. Survival After Exercise-Related Sudden Cardiac Arrest in Young Athletes: Can We Do Better? [Internet]. Vol. 11, Sports health. Sports Health; 2019 [cited 23 Oct 2020]. Available from: https://pubmed.ncbi.nlm.nih.gov/30204540/

9. Maron BJ, Thompson PD, Ackerman MJ, Balady G, Berger S, Cohen D, et al. Recommendations and Considerations Related to Preparticipation Screening for Cardiovascular Abnormalities in Competitive Athletes: 2007 Update. Circulation [Internet]. 27 March 2007 [cited 23 Oct 2020]; Available from: https://www.ahajournals.org/doi/abs/10.1161/CIRCULATIONAHA.107.181423

10. McKinney J, Velghe J, Fee J, Isserow S, Drezner JA. Defining Athletes and Exercisers. Am J Cardiol. 01 2019;123(3):532-5.

11. Caspersen CJ, Powell KE, Christenson GM. Physical activity, exercise, and physical fitness: definitions and distinctions for health-related research. Public Health Rep. 1985;100(2):126-31.

12. Tjønna AE, Stølen TO, Bye A, Volden M, Slørdahl SA, Odegård R, et al. Aerobic interval training reduces cardiovascular risk factors more than a multitreatment approach in overweight adolescents. Clin Sci (Lond). Feb 2009;116(4):317-26.

13. Schjerve IE, Tyldum GA, Tjønna AE, Stølen T, Loennechen JP, Hansen HEM, et al. Both aerobic endurance and strength training programmes improve cardiovascular health in obese adults. Clin Sci (Lond). Nov 2008;115(9):283-93.

14. Vanhees L, De Sutter J, GeladaS N, Doyle F, Prescott E, Cornelissen V, et al. Importance of characteristics and modalities of physical activity and exercise in defining the benefits to cardiovascular health within the general population: recommendations from the EACPR (Part I). Eur J Prev Cardiol. August 2012;19(4):670-86.

15. Shephard Roy J., Balady Gary J. Exercise as Cardiovascular Therapy. Circulation. 23 Feb 1999;99(7):963-72.

16. Lavie CJ, Thomas RJ, Squires RW, Allison TG, Milani RV. Exercise training and cardiac rehabilitation in primary and secondary prevention of coronary heart disease. Mayo Clin Proc. Apr 2009;84(4):373-83.

17. Franckowiak SC, Dobrosielski DA, Reilley SM, Walston JD, Andersen RE. Maximal heart rate prediction in adults that are overweight or obese. J Strength Cond Res. May 2011;25(5):1407-12.

18. Myers J, Hadley D, Oswald U, Bruner K, Kottman W, Hsu L, et al. Effects of exercise training on heart rate recovery in patients with chronic heart failure. Am Heart J. June 2007;153(6):1056-63.

19. Warburton DER, Nicol CW, Bredin SSD. Health benefits of physical activity: the evidence. CMAJ. March 14, 2006;174(6):801-9.

20. Pelliccia A, Sharma S, Gati S, Bäck M, Börjesson M, Caselli S, et al. 2020 ESC Guidelines on sports cardiology and exercise in patients with cardiovascular disease. European Heart Journal. 29 August 2020;ehaa605.

21. Anderson A, Forsyth A. Playing It Safe-BleedingDisorders, Sports and Exercise. New York, NY: National Hemophilia Foundation; 2017.

22. Mandsager K, Harb S, Cremer P, Phelan D, Nissen SE, Jaber W. Association of Cardiorespiratory Fitness With Long-term Mortality Among Adults Undergoing Exercise Treadmill Testing. JAMA Netw Open. 19 Oct 2018;1(6):e183605.

23. Shiroma EJ, Lee I-M. Physical activity and cardiovascular health: lessons learned from epidemiological studies across age, gender, and race/ethnicity. Circulation. August 17, 2010;122(7):743-52.

24. Radford NB, DeFina LF, Leonard D, Barlow CE, Willis BL, Gibbons LW, et al. Cardiorespiratory Fitness, Coronary Artery Calcium, and Cardiovascular Disease Events in a Cohort of Generally Healthy Middle-Age Men: Results From the Cooper Center Longitudinal Study. Circulation. 01 2018;137(18):1888-95.

25. Shah RV, Murthy VL, Colangelo LA, Reis J, Venkatesh BA, Sharma R, et al. Association of

Fitness in Young Adulthood With Survival and Cardiovascular Risk: The Coronary Artery Risk Development in Young Adults (CARDIA) Study. JAMA Intern Med. Jan 2016;176(1):87-95.

26. Hussain N, Gersh BJ, Gonzalez Carta K, Sydó N, Lopez-Jimenez F, Kopecky SL, et al. Impact of Cardiorespiratory Fitness on Frequency of Atrial Fibrillation, Stroke, and All-Cause Mortality. Am J Cardiol. 1 Jan 2018;121(1):41-9.

27. Juraschek SP, Blaha MJ, Whelton SP, Blumenthal R, Jones SR, Keteyian SJ, et al. Physical fitness and hypertension in a population at risk for cardiovascular disease: the Henry Ford Exerclse Testing (FIT) Project. J Am Heart Assoc. Dec 2014;3(6):e001268.

28. Juraschek SP, Blaha MJ, Blumenthal RS, Brawner C, Qureshi W, Keteyian SJ, et al. Cardiorespiratory fitness and incident diabetes: the FIT (Henry Ford Exerclse Testing) project. Diabetes Care. June 2015;38(6):1075-81.

29. Powell KE, King AC, Buchner DM, Campbell WW, DiPietro L, Erickson KI, et al. The Scientific Foundation for the Physical Activity Guidelines for Americans, 2nd Edition. J Phys Act Health. 17 Dec 2018;1-11.

30. Kyu HH, Bachman VF, Alexander LT, Mumford JE, Afshin A, Estep K, et al. Physical activity and risk of breast cancer, colon cancer, diabetes, ischemic heart disease, and ischemic stroke events: systematic review and dose-response meta-analysis for the Global Burden of Disease Study 2013. BMJ. 9 August 2016;354:i3857.

31. Haim M, Hoshen M, Reges O, Rabi Y, Balicer R, Leibowitz M. Prospective national study of the prevalence, incidence, management and outcome of a large contemporary cohort of patients with incident non-valvular atrial fibrillation. J Am Heart Assoc. 21 Jan 2015;4(1):e001486.

32. Chugh SS, Havmoeller R, Narayanan K, Singh D, Rienstra M, Benjamin EJ, et al. Worldwide epidemiology of atrial fibrillation: a Global Burden of Disease 2010 Study. Circulation. 25 Feb 2014;129(8):837-47.

33. Cushman M. Epidemiology and risk factors for venous thrombosis. Semin Hematol. Apr 2007;44(2):62-9.

34. Mont L, Sambola A, Brugada J, Vacca M, Marrugat J, Elosua R, et al. Long-lasting sport practice and lone atrial fibrillation. Eur Heart J. 1 March 2002;23(6):477-82.

35. Karjalainen J, Kujala UM, Kaprio J, Sarna S, Viitasalo M. Lone atrial fibrillation in vigorously exercising middle aged men: case-control study. BMJ. 13 June 1998;316(7147):1784-5.

36. Wilhelm M. Atrial fibrillation in endurance athletes: European Journal of Preventive Cardiology [Internet]. 30 Jan 2013 [cited 26 Oct 2020]; Available from: https://journals.sagepub.com/doi/10.1177/2047487313476414

37. Sanchis-Gomar F, Perez-Quilis C, Lippi G, Cervellin G, Leischik R, Löllgen H, et al. Atrial fibrillation in highly trained endurance athletes - Description of a syndrome. International Journal of Cardiology. 1 Jan 2017;226:11-20.

38. Myrstad M, Nystad W, Graff-Iversen S, Thelle DS, Stigum H, Aarønæs M, et al. Effect of Years of Endurance Exercise on Risk of Atrial Fibrillation and Atrial Flutter. The American Journal of Cardiology. 15 Oct 2014;114(8):1229-33.

39. Ofman P, Khawaja O, Rahilly-Tierney CR, Peralta A, Hoffmeister P, Reynolds MR, et al. Regular physical activity and risk of atrial fibrillation: a systematic review and meta-analysis. Circ Arrhythm Electrophysiol. Apr 2013;6(2):252-6.

40. Kwok CS, Anderson SG, Myint PK, Mamas MA, Loke YK. Physical activity and incidence of atrial fibrillation: A systematic review and meta-analysis. International Journal of Cardiology. 15 Dec 2014;177(2):467-76.

41. Abdulla J, Nielsen JR. Is the risk of atrial fibrillation higher in athletes than in the general population? A systematic review and meta-analysis. Europace. 1 Sep 2009;11(9):1156-9.

42. Aizer A, Gaziano JM, Cook NR, Manson JE, Buring JE, Albert CM. Relation of Vigorous Exercise to Risk of Atrial Fibrillation. The American Journal of Cardiology. June 1, 2009;103(11):1572-7.

43. Andersen K, Farahmand B, Ahlbom A, Held C, Ljunghall S, Michaëlsson K, et al. Risk of arrhythmias in 52 755 long-distance cross-country skiers: a cohort study. European Heart Journal. 14 Dec 2013;34(47):3624-31.

44. Thelle DS, Selmer R, Gjesdal K, Sakshaug S, Jugessur A, Graff-Iversen S, et al. Resting heart rate and physical activity as risk factors for lone atrial fibrillation: a prospective study of 309,540 men and women. Heart. 1 Dec 2013;99(23):1755-60.

45. Nielsen JR, Wachtell K, Abdulla J. The Relationship Between Physical Activity and Risk of Atrial Fibrillation-A Systematic Review and Meta-Analysis. J Atr Fibrillation [Internet]. Feb 12, 2013 [cited Oct 26, 2020];5(5). Available from: https://www.ncbi.nlm.nih.gov/pmc/articles/PMC5153110/

46. Mont L, Investigators on behalf of the G (Grup I de R en FA, Tamborero D, Investigators on behalf of the G (Grup I de R en FA, Elosua R, Investigators on behalf of the G (Grup I de R en FA, et al. Physical activity, height, and left atrial size are independent risk factors for lone atrial fibrillation in middle-aged healthy individuals. Europace. 1 Jan 2008;10(1):15-20.

47. Mozaffarian D, Furberg CD, Psaty BM, Siscovick D. Physical activity and incidence of atrial fibrillation in older adults: the cardiovascular health study. Circulation. 19 August 2008;118(8):800-7.

48. Mohanty S, Mohanty P, Tamaki M, Natale V, Gianni C, Trivedi C, et al. Differential Association of Exercise Intensity With Risk of Atrial Fibrillation in Men and Women: Evidence from a Meta- Analysis. J Cardiovasc Electrophysiol. 2016;27(9):1021-9.

49. Coumel P. Paroxysmal Atrial Fibrillation: A Disorder of Autonomic Tone? European Heart Journal. 1 Apr 1994;15(suppl_A):9-16.

50. Aubert AE, Seps B, Beckers F. Heart Rate Variability in Athletes. Sports Med. 1 Oct 2003;33(12):889-919.

51. Elliott AD, Mahajan R, Lau DH, Sanders P. Atrial Fibrillation in Endurance Athletes: From Mechanism to Management. Cardiology Clinics. Nov 1, 2016;34(4):567-78.

52. Guasch E, Benito B, Qi X, Cifelli C, Naud P, Shi Y, et al. Atrial Fibrillation Promotion by Endurance Exercise: Demonstration and Mechanistic Exploration in an Animal Model. Journal of the American College of Cardiology. 2 Jul 2013;62(1):68-77.

53. Nattel S, Harada M. Atrial Remodeling and Atrial Fibrillation: Recent Advances and Translational Perspectives. Journal of the American College of Cardiology. June 10, 2014;63(22):2335-45.

54. Estes NAM, Madias C. Atrial Fibrillation in Athletes: A Lesson in the Virtue of Moderation. JACC Clin Electrophysiol. 2017;3(9):921-8.

55. Fragakis N, Vicedomini G, Pappone C. Endurance Sport Activity and Risk of Atrial Fibrillation - Epidemiology, Proposed Mechanisms and Management. Arrhythm Electrophysiol Rev. May 2014;3(1):15-9.

56. Sharma S, Merghani A, Mont L. Exercise and the heart: the good, the bad, and the ugly. European Heart Journal. 14 June 2015;36(23):1445-53.

57. Wernhart S, Halle M. Atrial fibrillation and long-term sports practice: epidemiology and mechanisms. Clin Res Cardiol. 1 May 2015;104(5):369-79.

58. Turagam MK, Velagapudi P, Kocheril AG. Atrial Fibrillation in Athletes. The American Journal of Cardiology. 15 Jan 2012;109(2):296-302.

59. Carpenter A, Frontera A, Bond R, Duncan E, Thomas G. Vagal atrial fibrillation: What is it and should we treat it? International Journal of Cardiology. 15 Dec 2015;201:415-21.

60. Coumel P. Paroxysmal Atrial Fibrillation: A Disorder of Autonomic Tone? European Heart Journal. 1 Apr 1994;15(suppl_A):9-16.

61. Grundvold Irene, Skretteberg Per Torger, Liestøl Knut, Erikssen Gunnar, Engeseth Kristian, Gjesdal Knut, et al. Low Heart Rates Predict Incident Atrial Fibrillation in Healthy Middle-Aged Men. Circulation: Arrhythmia and Electrophysiology. August 1, 2013;6(4):726-31.

62. Kirchhof P, Benussi S, Kotecha D, Ahlsson A, Atar D, Casadei B, et al. 2016 ESC Guidelines for the management of atrial fibrillation developed in collaboration with EACTS. European Heart Journal. 7 Oct 2016;37(38):2893-962.

63. Lip GYH, Nieuwlaat R, Pisters R, Lane DA, Crijns HJGM. Refining clinical risk stratification for predicting stroke and thromboembolism in atrial fibrillation using a novel risk factor-based approach: the euro heart survey on atrial fibrillation. Chest. Feb 2010;137(2):263-72.

64. Hindricks G, Potpara T, Dagres N, Arbelo E, Bax JJ, Blomström-Lundqvist C, et al. 2020 ESC Guidelines for the diagnosis and management of atrial fibrillation developed in collaboration with the European Association of Cardio-Thoracic Surgery (EACTS). European Heart Journal. 29 August 2020;ehaa612.

65. Khan IA. Atrial stunning: basics and clinical considerations. Int J Cardiol. Dec 2003;92(2-3):113-28.

66. Hoogsteen J, Schep G, Van Hemel NM, Van Der Wall EE. Paroxysmal atrial fibrillation in male endurance athletes. A 9-year follow up. Europace. May 2004;6(3):222-8.

67. Baldesberger S, Bauersfeld U, Candinas R, Seifert B, Zuber M, Ritter M, et al. Sinus node disease and arrhythmias in the long-term follow-up of former professional cyclists. Eur Heart J. Jan 2008;29(1):71-8.

68. Heidbüchel H, Anné W, Willems R, Adriaenssens B, Van de Werf F, Ector H. Endurance sports is a risk factor for atrial fibrillation after ablation for atrial flutter. Int J Cardiol. 8 Feb 2006;107(1):67-72.

69. van Stralen KJ, Le Cessie S, Rosendaal FR, Doggen CJM. Regular sports activities decrease the risk of venous thrombosis. J Thromb Haemost. Nov 2007;5(11):2186-92.

70. Fink ML, Stoneman PD. Deep Vein Thrombosis in an Athletic Military Cadet. J Orthop Sports Phys Ther. 1 Sep 2006;36(9):686-97.

71. Bishop M, Astolfi M, Padegimas E, DeLuca P, Hammoud S. Venous Thromboembolism Within Professional American Sport Leagues. Orthopaedic Journal of Sports Medicine. 1 Dec 2017;5(12):2325967117745530.

72. Gunga H-C, Kirsch K, Beneke R, Böning D, Hopfenmüller W, Leithäuser R, et al. Markers of coagulation, fibrinolysis and angiogenesis after strenuous short-term exercise (Wingate-test) in male subjects of varying fitness levels. Int J Sports Med. Oct 2002;23(7):495-9.

73. El-Sayed MS, El-Sayed Ali Z, Ahmadizad S. Exercise and Training Effects on Blood Haemostasis in Health and Disease. Sports Med. 1 March 2004;34(3):181-200.

74. Tao K, Davenport M. Deep Venous Thromboembolism in a Triathlete. The Journal of Emergency Medicine. 1 Apr 2010;38(3):351-3.

75. Zadow EK, Adams MJ, Kitic CM, Wu SSX, Fell JW. Acquired and Genetic Thrombotic Risk Factors in the Athlete. Semin Thromb Hemost. Nov 2018;44(8):723-33.

76. Hull Claire M., Harris Julia A. Venous Thromboembolism and Marathon Athletes. Circulation. 1 Dec 2013;128(25):e469-71.

77. Heil J, Miesbach W, Vogl T, Bechstein WO, Reinisch A. Deep Vein Thrombosis of the Upper Extremity. Dtsch Arztebl Int. 7 Apr 2017;114(14):244-9.

78. Sajid MS, Ahmed N, Desai M, Baker D, Hamilton G. Upper Limb Deep Vein Thrombosis: A Literature Review to Streamline the Protocol for Management. AHA. 2007;118(1):10-8.

79. Huang C-Y, Wu Y-H, Yeh I-J, Chen Y-Y, Kung F-Y. Spontaneous bilateral subclavian vein thrombosis in a 40-year-old man: A case report. Medicine. Apr 2018;97(15):e0327.

80. Illig KA, Doyle AJ. A comprehensive review of Paget-Schroetter syndrome. Journal of Vascular Surgery. June 1, 2010;51(6):1538-47.

81. Alla VM, Natarajan N, Kaushik M, Warrier R, Nair CK. Paget-schroetter syndrome: review of pathogenesis and treatment of effort thrombosis. West J Emerg Med. Sep 2010;11(4):358-62.

82. Naeem M, Soares G, Ahn S, Murphy TP. Paget-Schroetter syndrome: A review and Algorithm (WASPS-IR): Phlebology [Internet]. Feb 11, 2015 [cited Oct 27, 2020]; Available from: https://journals.sagepub.com/doi/10.1177/0268355514568534

83. Altintaş F, Uluçay Ç. Deep Vein Thrombosis in Athletes: Prevention and Treatment. In: Doral MN, editor. Sports Injuries: Prevention, Diagnosis, Treatment and Rehabilitation [Internet]. Berlin, Heidelberg: Springer; 2012 [cited 27 Oct 2020]. p. 1065-71. Disponible sur: https://doi.org/10.1007/978-3-642-15630-4_141

84. Yim ES, Corrado G. Ultrasound in Athletes: Emerging Techniques in Point-of-Care Practice. Current Sports Medicine Reports. Dec 2012;11(6):298-303.

85. Kearon C, Akl EA. Duration of anticoagulant therapy for deep vein thrombosis and pulmonary embolism. Blood. March 20, 2014;123(12):1794-801.

86. Kearon C, Akl EA, Ornelas J, Blaivas A, Jimenez D, Bounameaux H, et al. Antithrombotic Therapy for VTE Disease: CHEST Guideline and Expert Panel Report. Chest. Feb 2016;149(2):315-52.

87. Moffatt K, Silberberg PJ, Gnarra DJ. Pulmonary embolism in an adolescent soccer player: a case report. Med Sci Sports Exerc. June 2007;39(6):899-902.

88. Croyle PH, Place RA, Hilgenberg AD. Massive Pulmonary Embolism in a High School Wrestler. JAMA. Feb 23, 1979;241(8):827-8.

89. Kearon C, Akl EA, Comerota AJ, Prandoni P, Bounameaux H, Goldhaber SZ, et al. Antithrombotic Therapy for VTE Disease. Chest. Feb 2012;141(2 Suppl):e419S-e494S.

90. Di Nisio M, Wichers IM, Middeldorp S. Treatment for superficial thrombophlebitis of the leg. Cochrane Database Syst Rev. 30 Apr 2013;(4):CD004982.

91. Hill SL, Hancock DH, Webb TL. Thrombophlebitis of the great saphenous vein-- recommendations for treatment. Phlebology. 2008;23(1):35-9.

92. Yeh CH, Hogg K, Weitz JI. Overview of the new oral anticoagulants: opportunities and challenges. Arterioscler Thromb Vasc Biol. May 2015;35(5):1056-65.

93. Ferri N, Corsini A. Nuovi anticoagulanti orali: considerazioni di farmacologia clinica [Internet]. Vol. 16, Giornale Italiano di Cardiologia. 2015 [cited 29 Oct 2020]. p. 3-16. Available from: /

94. Leow AS-T, Sia C-H, Tan BY-Q, Loh JP-Y. A meta-summary of case reports of non-vitamin K antagonist oral anticoagulant use in patients with left ventricular thrombus. J Thromb Thrombolysis. Jul 2018;46(1):68-73.

95. Wang Y, Bajorek B. New oral anticoagulants in practice: pharmacological and practical considerations. Am J Cardiovasc Drugs. June 2014;14(3):175-89.

96. Gong IY, Kim RB. Importance of pharmacokinetic profile and variability as determinants of dose and response to dabigatran, rivaroxaban, and apixaban. Can J Cardiol. Jul 2013;29(7 Suppl):S24- 33.

97. Sairaku A, Nakano Y, Onohara Y, Hironobe N, Matsumura H, Shimizu W, et al. Residual anticoagulation activity in atrial fibrillation patients with temporarily interrupted direct oral anticoagulants: Comparisons across 4 drugs. Thromb Res. Nov 2019;183:119-23.

98. Mega JL, Braunwald E, Wiviott SD, Bassand J-P, Bhatt DL, Bode C, et al. Rivaroxaban in patients with a recent acute coronary syndrome. N Engl J Med. 2012 Jan 5;366(1):9-19.

99. Eikelboom JW, Connolly SJ, Bosch J, Dagenais GR, Hart RG, Shestakovska O, et al. Rivaroxaban with or without Aspirin in Stable Cardiovascular Disease. New England Journal of Medicine. 5 Oct 2017;377(14):1319-30.

100.	Maron BJ, Zipes DP. Introduction: eligibility recommendations for competitive athletes with cardiovascular abnormalities-general considerations. J Am Coll Cardiol. 19 Apr 2005;45(8):1318-21.

101.	Maron BJ, Zipes DP, Kovacs RJ. Eligibility and Disqualification Recommendations for Competitive Athletes With Cardiovascular Abnormalities: Preamble, Principles, and General Considerations: A Scientific Statement From the American Heart Association and American College of Cardiology. J Am Coll Cardiol. 1 Dec 2015;66(21):2343-9.

102.	Panno VA, Gulizia M, Colivicchi F, Lenarda AD, Casasco M, Zeppilli P, et al. COMPOSIZIONE COMITATO COCIS. 2017;232.

103.	Berkowitz JN, Moll S. Athletes and blood clots: individualized, intermittent anticoagulation management. J Thromb Haemost. 2017;15(6):1051-4.

104.	Samuelson BT, Cuker A, Siegal DM, Crowther M, Garcia DA. Laboratory Assessment of the Anticoagulant Activity of Direct Oral Anticoagulants: A Systematic Review. Chest. Jan 2017;151(1):127-38.

105.	Moll S, Berkowitz JN, Miars CW. Elite athletes and anticoagulant therapy: an intermittent dosing strategy. Hematology Am Soc Hematol Educ Program. 30 2018;2018(1):412-7.

106.	Chan NC, Hirsh J, Ginsberg JS, Eikelboom JW. Real-world variability in dabigatran levels in patients with atrial fibrillation: reply. Journal of Thrombosis and Haemostasis. 2015;13(6):1168-9.

107.	Sanna GD, Gabrielli E, De Vito E, Nusdeo G, Prisco D, Parodi G. Atrial fibrillation in athletes: From epidemiology to treatment in the novel oral anticoagulants era. Journal of Cardiology. 1 Oct 2018;72(4):269-76.

108.	January CT, Wann LS, Alpert JS, Calkins H, Cigarroa JE, Cleveland JC, et al. 2014 AHA/ACC/HRS guideline for the management of patients with atrial fibrillation: executive summary: a report of the American College of Cardiology/American Heart Association Task Force on practice guidelines and the Heart Rhythm Society. Circulation. 2 Dec 2014;130(23):2071-104.

109.	Heidbüchel H, Panhuyzen-Goedkoop N, Corrado D, Hoffmann E, Biffi A, Delise P, et al. Recommendations for participation in leisure-time physical activity and competitive sports in patients with arrhythmias and potentially arrhythmogenic conditions Part I: Supraventricular arrhythmias and pacemakers. Eur J Cardiovasc Prev Rehabil. August 2006;13(4):475-84.

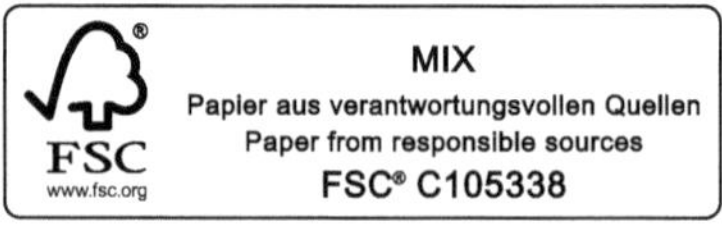

Printed by Books on Demand GmbH, Norderstedt / Germany